WELCOME

So, why write a book on Grandma's Personal Training?

We see personal training for Over 50s or for older people, but we don't see books and programmes directly written for a grandma or indeed for a granddad! This is where this lack of information stops, because, if you are a grandma or granddad, this information is for you.

As we become older, as we know, if you have been employed or have worked for yourself in your own business, you may have looked forward to your day of retirement. At that point in time, retirement seems to be a yearning and a time of change. Change is good for the human body and brain, but if that change incorporates stopping or totally stopping, then the deterioration of health may accelerate, this is not what retirement is about!

Retirement is a time to develop new skills, find new interests and to start to grow in both mind and body but in a new way that has not been available to you before. Many people become so busy in their jobs or bringing up a family, making sure that all is working well in the home, but they forget about who they are and what life has in store once they start to think differently!

I'm a mum, grandmother and have been waiting since I was seven years old to start my new career in writing. The writing is now into its twenty-sixth year and still I'm loving every word I put onto a page, but to write, I need to keep my brain, mind, and body in good working condition. If I was to stop what I'm doing, then I would not be writing this book with you in mind.

To retire and then STOP is a way to sickness and a shorter life span, and that is not what most people want. Having said that, as life goes on, and life still has its hurdles, if retired, we can easily slip into an abyss of depression or develop negative thinking which then leads to negative habits and negative outcomes; this is not a recipe for a healthy retirement, it is a recipe for self-decline.

Working in a regularly paid job, prior to retirement, regardless of the 'humdrum' of the job, gives us a sense of purpose and worth, and when we retire, that purpose has suddenly gone from our lives. In retirement, we may think that it's now 'our time' and can do exactly what we want to do and move into the 'do nothing' stage of life! If this applies to you, one day, you may wake up, and fill totally unfulfilled, have a low sense of worth and feel thoroughly miserable, this is now going to change.

IN THE BEGINNING – THIS IS ALL ABOUT YOU

Spending time on yourself is not selfish, it is your right to take some quality time out each week and to do the activities that are going to keep you, not only healthier, but safe. I say safe, because when your body moves easier, your reaction time becomes quicker, your brain can think sharply and your everyday existence becomes happier, life is no longer a chore, mundane jobs become easier to face, and we seem to do those jobs faster than we previously did. So, there are many benefits from doing a few easy and simple exercises every other or each day!

Instead of taking a fast, let's get this done, we are going to get to know each other and that starts me saying to you, 'Hello, it's lovely to see you and thank you for joining me.' We are also going to start by taking each day, one at a time.

You may wish to read the book, and think about the changes you want to make, that is fine, because many people like to take their time before their mind is ready for change and indeed, ready to do some muscle and body exercises.

Changing from possibly being overtaken by the feelings that, 'everyday life is a challenge and too hard', to the thoughts, 'OK, yes, I will take that on, I can do that...' may take some energy, but making the decision to change can reap many rewards, including feeling good about yourself, and being glad you are the person you are.

I not only love to write, but I used to love to paint large pictures of flowers. For many years, about thirteen in all, I hadn't picked up a paint brush or done anything creative other than write!
The writing, though it is my passion, is very demanding, very mentally restrictive and can totally absorb my life. As we know,

too much of a good thing, can leave us mentally and physically depleted of energy. I don't know where the idea of memory came from, but only recently, I decided to 'paint again' and this I have been doing. I now turn the computer off at about five-o'clock pm and do not touch the keyboard until the next day. I then have a light dinner and paint for a couple of hours. This new regime of working for me, has given me such a new empowerment in painting but it could only happen through making a determined choice.

The other hobby I've taken up and to allow me to write this book, I have started working with a personal exercise trainer. So, it is my intention to become your personal trainer over the time of you reading and enjoying this new part of your life. Please remember, you are doing this for you. This journey is about you, not me.

Having said the above, I will hasten to add here, as the author of the book, 'Devils In Our Food', I will also be speaking about the food you eat. Of course, you always have the choice to read, listen or take notice.

More than any other purpose, importantly, you will need to enjoy your exercise journey.

Published by How2Books
Under licence from MSI Ltd, Australia
Company Registration No: 96963518255
NSW, Australia

See our website: www.how2books.com.au
Or contact by email: sales@how2books.com.au
Covers and Copyright owned by MSI, Australia

MSI acknowledges the author and images, text and photographs used in this book.

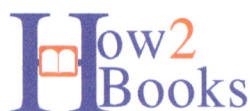

How2
Books

CONTENTS

PAGE

MODULE ONE
GETTING READY FOR THE EXERCISE JOURNEY
BE READY AND WHAT TO WEAR – TALKING ABOUT
YOU, ARM AND HEAD MOVEMENTS   1

MODULE TWO
BREATHING – IT IS THE MOST IMPORTANT PART
OF YOUR EXERCISE JOURNEY – HEAD EXERCISES
AND WRIST MOVEMENTS   20

MODULE THREE
LET'S TALK ABOUT YOUR BRAIN AND THE FOOD
YOU EAT...! EXERCISING YOUR LEGS, ANKLES
AND FEET   27

MODULE FOUR
THE MOLECULES IN YOUR FOOD AND DRINK –
KNEE LIFTS AND MORE LEG EXERCISES   45

MODULE FIVE
THE BENEFITS OF HAVING PURE GELATINE AND
MARROW BONE IN THE HUMAN DIET – USING YOUR
QUADS TO BETTER HEALTH - GLUTE BRIDGING AND
STRENGTHENING YOUR LOWER BODY   58

MODULE ONE - GETTING READY FOR THE EXERCISE JOURNEY
BE READY AND WHAT TO WEAR

Let's have some fun. When we think of exercising, we think of pain and hurt and yet, it shouldn't be like that. We are going to put some fun into the exercises we learn.

REMEMBER, TO START SLOWLY, BE CONSISTENT, YOU ARE BUILDING MUSCLE MASS AND BODY STRENGTH. You may not have exercised for some time, so please be kind to yourself.

1) To begin, put some moderate beat music on so that you have a rhythm to work with, but keep the music low.

As we become older, we need to be conscious that our body, though older, still needs to be looked after and loved. Keeping fit is just one way, we can show our body and brain that we are taking care of it.

Let's start at the beginning. You will need some comfortable clothing and secure shoes. Do not exercise in shoes that are likely to come off your feet or uncomfortable.

So,

a) Wear supporting shoes.
b) Wear comfortable clothing that feels nice to wear.

c) Keep some fresh water handy so that you can sip as you go – not too much, just moisten your mouth from time to time.

d) Remove any mats, rugs, or trip hazards from the floor. Only exercise on a secure surface.

e) If needed, use a kitchen, bathroom, or an extremely sturdy bench or table to use as a security base to do your exercises. Do not rely on any bench or surface that does not feel comfortable or is loose to the touch, remember, you are relying on the strength of the base you are holding on to!

f) Once you are ready, we will start.

THE BENEFITS OF EXERCISE TO YOUR BRAIN, MIND AND BODY

As we become older, it's not only important to do exercises but it's important to know what exercises are best for you! There are many factors to think about, factors include your lifestyle, and physical activity.

If you have health conditions, it is a matter of finding the exercises that work for you. If you want to exercise but are concerned about what exercises are right, please talk to your doctor, or do the exercises in this book that feel right for you.

Doing regular exercises helps with many health conditions, such as heart problems, diabetes (type 1 and 2), asthma, arthritis, osteoporosis, Parkinson's disease, dementia, or other health concerns.

Include, not only the exercises in this book, but walking, swimming, tennis, or activities that best suit you and your health.

Just a small increase in physical activity improves such conditions as high blood pressure, helps in the maintenance of weight, it reduces the risk of falls and injury, it gives more energy to your overall body and how you feel; improves sleep, will reduce stress and anxiety, improves your concentration and your mental health.

Age should not be a barrier to exercising. Some different activities that help to keep you fit, include cleaning, mopping, and vacuuming the house. Other fun activities are dancing, tai-chi, bowls, stretching and yoga.

Exercises help in building muscle body strength, keeping your brain healthy, which includes keeping your mind in good condition and supports you in your balance as you live the life you want to live.

Do not rush your exercises. When starting, only do the exercises your body can cope with. Please remember, if your body hasn't been worked for some time, it will go through a sense of shock, or a 'wake-up' call because you are now in the control seat of your brain and you are the one that is not going to be dictated to.

A little further on in the book, I speak about your brain, and it is a very obedient servant to you. If you give your brain the order, it will deliver. So, please remember, as you are changing and want to develop your health and wellbeing regime, there may be a certain resistance from the command centre in your brain because you are now taking charge.

Through life, you or we can develop bad habits, and some bad habits interfere with your wellbeing, like watching too much television than is good for you or eating an unhealthy diet! All actions which interfere with your health are doing so because in the beginning, you have given your brain the permission to accept that bad habit in the first place...!

Now, things are different, you are going to make the difference because you are making the choices to change to a healthy, maybe older person, who wants to maintain a sense of wellbeing, independence, and the enjoyment of life.

MODULE ONE CONTINUED
STARTING FROM SCRATCH – TALKING ABOUT YOU – ARM AND HEAD MOVEMENT EXERCISES

In this module you will learn:

- ✓ Getting to know your personality.
- ✓ The power of water and its therapy.
- ✓ The benefits of moving your upper body, exercising, and moving your arms.
- ✓ How exercise benefits your overall health and wellbeing.

Everything we say or do, starts with us thinking about the process before the action is taken and that is why, it is important for you to make the choices to do the exercises.

Remembering choices are made in your brain in your head, and you have the choice to work towards your wellbeing.

Many times, when you want to make positive changes in your lifestyle, you may experience your inner voice saying, 'No, I can't do that today!' 'It's too hard, no, I'll do that tomorrow...!' When you get caught up in this type of thinking, you may be going on a slippery slide and mentally downhill. Many of these negative thoughts are indeed bad habits that we create within our own thinking, and once they are created, they can be extremely difficult to remove.

I too, have had and do have, these own inner struggles where one part of my mind doesn't want to do something, and I had previously planned to do that something..., then my mental wellbeing is thrown into disarray because I have allowed myself to become conflicted, that then causes stress and has all sorts of negative outcomes on my body and mind, and then on my health and positive wellbeing.

Now, let's take this information a little further, once understood, other information will make more sense.

Eric Berne, psychiatrist, please don't let his title put you off, he makes a lot of sense. Berne, identified, we each have three different personality states; each personality works within us each moment of every day:

1) *The Adult Personality State.* When you are in this personality, you are firm, yet fair and when you make up your mind to do something, you do it. In this personality state, you are understanding but take a mature approach to life and the issues you are facing. You are 'matter of fact' not cruel, just honest and to the point. You may also like time to think things through, but once your mind is made up, you work towards your commitment, in this case, it would be committing to activities that support you in your mental health and your body's wellbeing.

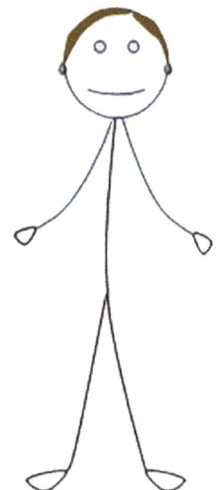

2) *The Parent Personality State.* When you are in this personality, you are authoritarian, and may not listen to reason, and be content with your own point of view!

When your Parent personality has dominance in your thinking, it can interfere with the goals you have set yourself.

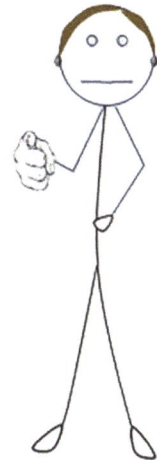

Within the Parent Personality, you may also give your alternative views to other people of 'why' you and they should not exercise. The Parent personality state wants to be heard and this personality thrives on other people agreeing. If you feel this confusion in your thinking, try to think about your Adult personality and the commitment to the plans you have made.

3) *The Child Personality State.* When you are in your Child personality, you may do everything you can think of to sabotage your exercise programme. You can make excuses not to get off the couch, not get out of bed at the appropriate time! If you had decided to do the exercise programme with other people, you may make excuses not to meet up. You can indeed have a two-year-old tantrum within your head, you may also feel you want to stamp your feet or scream because when a two-year-old does not get their own way, this is sometimes the behaviour they display!

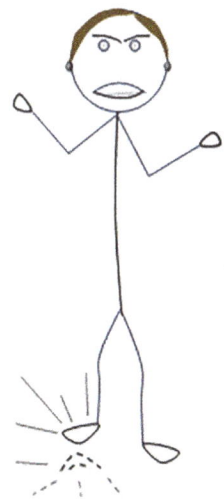

Bad habits need to be broken to allow you to become healthy. From observation, we may develop bad habits when we are in the Child personality state; this state is an 'instant gratification' state and wants instant rewards. In this state, long-term objectives and goals are not set; the work associated with getting to great and positive achievements or outcomes does not happen if permanently thinking negative thoughts! If this happens, you will need to be strong. When bad habits have developed and bad habits, because your personality states may have been out of control, these bad habits are reluctant to give in to change and the positive changes you are making.

However, by determination and persistence, even the worst and most destructive habits can be broken and breaking bad habits comes from working with your Adult personality state.

To quickly mention here, we need at different times to work with all three personality states, life would be boring if we only worked continuously with the Adult personality state.

As a grandmother, I like to work with the granddaughters when we sit and paint or make jewellery together or if I'm reading a story, there are parts of all three personalities that need to be working at these times.

It is important to get to know your own personality states because by doing so, you are in control of the actions you take and the words you speak, and that makes you a powerful, well-balanced, human being. By achieving this control, you can climb almost impossible heights with goals, achieve what you may have thought you could not achieve, and so much more.

I also find, by working quietly and within my head, I can achieve so much more, like writing the books I write, paint the pictures I want to paint, and achieve far reaching goals that are my own goals and belong to nobody else but me! My goals do not hurt any other person but give me great satisfaction when they are achieved. If you like, I don't let anybody pull or manipulate those emotional strings that so many people are controlled by. I now live life according to my terms and not those of other people!

So, by getting my head sorted out, it allows me to move on and enjoy every moment of every day.

With this new beginning you are going to have some fun. To begin each day, the night before, you need to write down your goals for the following day. I do this every day, even if the goals are not related to exercise or the work I do. If I don't write my goals down, and leave them in my thoughts inside my head, many times, those goals are not achieved the following day and I end up feeling frustrated with myself and that leads to stress and stress I don't need as a seventy-seven-year-old, grandmother...!

TAKING ONE DAY ONE STEP AT A TIME

Before starting to exercise each day, I start, first with a positive mindset. This mindset is put into reality the day before by writing down the jobs or exercises I want to do the following day. By writing your goals down, you are indeed making a 'mental contract' with yourself; these contracts are powerful tools when you want to achieve goals.

In many instances, when I've been teaching, any subject, including psychology, I've asked my students to write down their goals and in doing so, they are giving their brain an order, and your brain being the obedient servant that it is, will obey you. Having said that, if you sabotage your goals by giving your brain a counter-order of not to do the goals you have previously meant to do, you too, are responsible for the destruction you are causing yourself!

You may wish to start your exercises by sitting down on a chair, if you can stand, it is better to do so, as you maintain your body's physical balance.

To exercise, and not hurt yourself, you need to prepare your body and mind. I do this by having a warm shower before doing any fitness or exercise programme.

An added advantage to any wellbeing programmes is to have your 'head in the right place', and softly running water over your head can help to create the right 'head space' to achieve the maximum benefits from the exercises you are about to do.

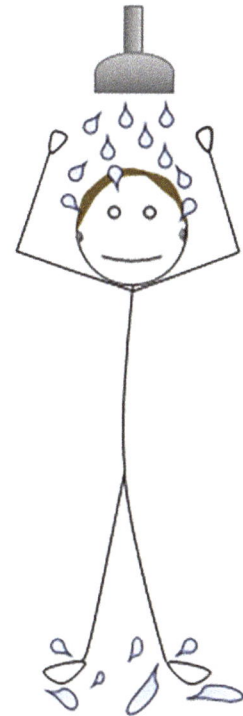

When you feel the benefits of the running water over your head and body, the water's energy will support your sense of wellbeing when you start your exercises. By adding this small action to your daily regime, even if not exercising, it will add to your health, lessen any form of negative stress, and give you a sense of personal worth because you are investing in 'you'...

Many older people may feel embarrassed about exercising, there is no need for this, if this is you, 'STOP' right now, you are worthy of the investment you are making in yourself. Embarrassment may lead to a destructive attitude which may limit personal growth and achievement.

YOUR WELLBEING

As we become older, regardless of status, life can offer up some difficult times! I once, would have my shower, apply moisturiser to all my body before starting to limber up for my exercises!

Through many of life's traumas, we simply want to get through the day, and cannot wait for an awful time to pass; regardless of the outcome...! It is at this time, we go into 'existence' mode, or 'survival' mode, we do the essential to keep ourselves moving forward, but that is all we do!

Things are going to change right now. Once you have had your shower and feel good about you. It is time to apply moisturiser to your body, arms, legs, feet, face, and hands. This recognition to your body allows your brain to record the good steps you are doing to keep you well and healthy.

HORMONES

I have written many books about hormones, in fact, I find hormones so incredibly interesting that they deserve far more recognition to the human body, than they are given within the public consciousness and awareness. Hormones are your body's messengers and work within every part of your body, and some are connected and live inside your brain. They let you know when you have an itch, when you are hungry, when to go to bed, when you fall in love, when you feel anger and so much more.

By taking care of your body through having a relaxing shower, then applying moisturiser to your body and face, you are indeed sending good messages, through your hormone messengers, to your brain.

ARM MOVEMENTS AND ROTATIONS

The first exercise after your shower is to start to get your upper body moving, this includes your arms and neck.

Try to do your exercises while your body is still warm from your shower.

Rotate your arm in a backward motion five times, if you can manage ten, then do ten backward motions.

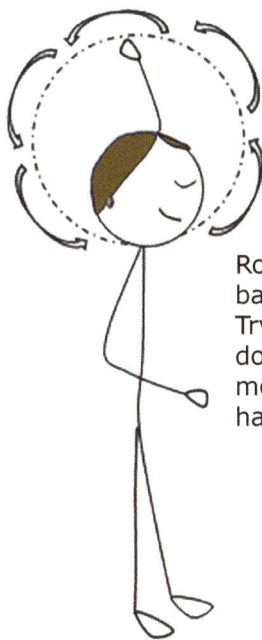

Rotating your arm in a back circular motion. Try to count to ten. Or do the number of arm movements you feel happy with.

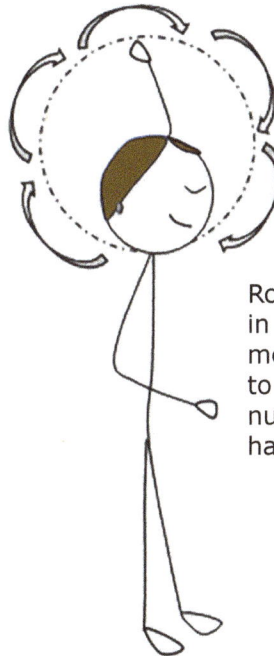

Rotating your arm in a front circular motion. Try to count to ten. Or do the number you feel happy with.

These are just simple exercises to limber you up and to get you into the habit of feeling good.

Once you have rotated your arm in the backward movement, then come forwards in a similar circular motion. Once completed, follow the same exercise with your other arm.

After completing the previous exercises, take a short 30 second break and then move onto the next exercise, which is slowly moving your arms above your head.

ARM AND HAND UPWARD STRETCHING

Starting with either your left or right arm, reach high above your head and stretch as high and into the air as you can. 'STRETCH', 'STRETCH', 'STRETCH', reaching high, and up to the sky. Once you are satisfied with your effort, bring your arm down and then bring the other arm up and do the same as previously done. Remembering to, 'STRETCH', 'STRETCH', 'STRETCH', reaching high and up to the sky...!

Also, please think, you may not have done any exercises for a while, please only do the exercises you feel comfortable doing. Having said this, please also think about your Adult personality state and be aware of not sabotaging your goals.

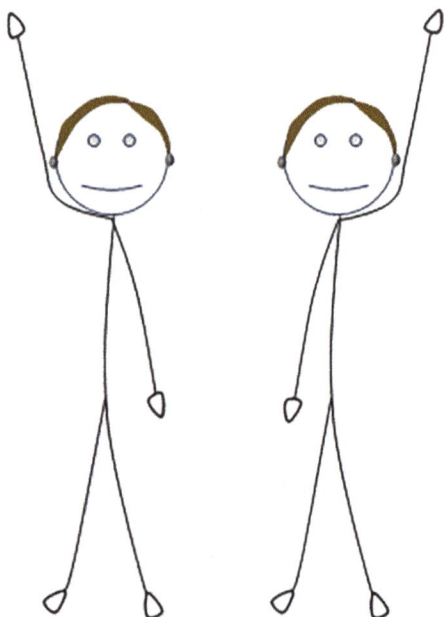

Keeping your arms as straight as possible, reach for the sky, first your left, then your right. Always remember to keep your feet straight in front of you.

As your body starts to loosen up, you will feel the relief in your shoulders and neck.

14

Now, because you want the maximum benefit from the exercises you are doing, bring both arms up into the air and above your head. If you can, touch, or clasp your hands together, count to five or ten.

Remembering to, **'STRETCH', 'STRETCH', 'STRETCH',** reaching high and up to the sky…!

Rest for thirty seconds, then raise your arms up and over your head as in the last exercise but move, at your own speed from side to side; don't overdo it but feel the tension in your body as you move.

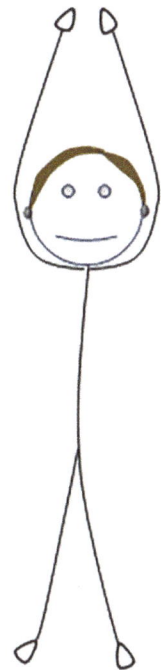

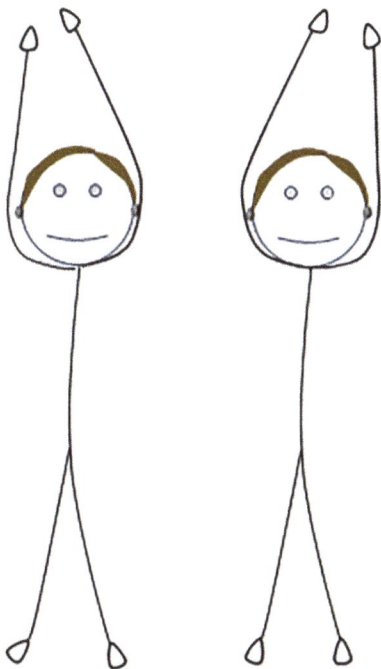

As you stretch from your left to the right, your body will move in a different way, possibly, now as it has not done for some time. Be gentle with yourself with your exercises but be firm and determined.

When you feel ready, stop, relax for thirty seconds and we'll move onto your head and neck.

I have found, when my neck becomes stiff or my shoulders seem fixed, my general health seems to decline. By keeping this part of my body flexible, I can think clearly, I feel able to cope with everyday situations more readily and overall, I feel healthy and able to take on new challenges.

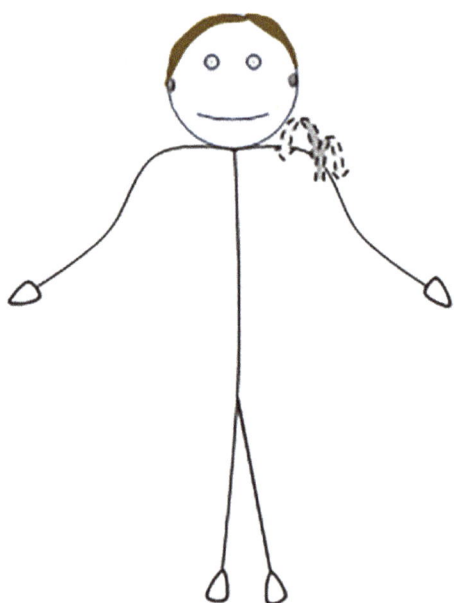

ROLLING YOUR SHOULDERS

Rolling your shoulder forward for five and then rolling it backwards for five, then exercise the opposite shoulder in the same way.

As you roll your shoulders, you will also exercise you arm socket, so, this exercise offers a double benefit.

Always do exercises using the same number of movements for each part of you, on every part of your body. Do not favour one part of your body over another part, even if the exercise is easy on one side or part and difficult on the other side or part; try to treat both the same.

When you have completed your shoulder exercises, take a short thirty-second break, sip some water, and make yourself ready to continue with your exercise regime.

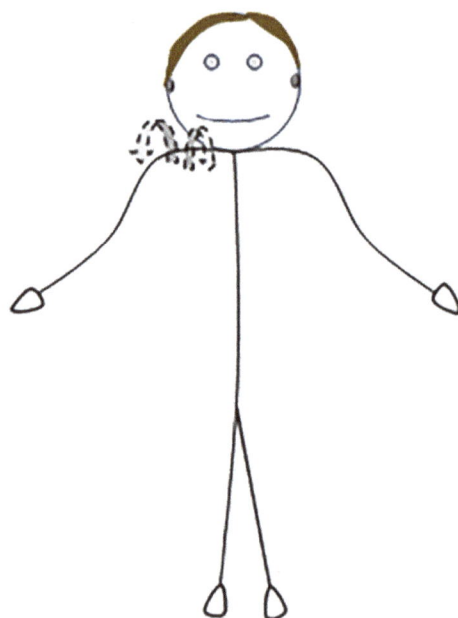

BOTH ARM ROTATIONS

Now that you have started moving and are feeling confident with the exercises you are doing, let's give your arms a good workout.

1)

2)

3)

4)

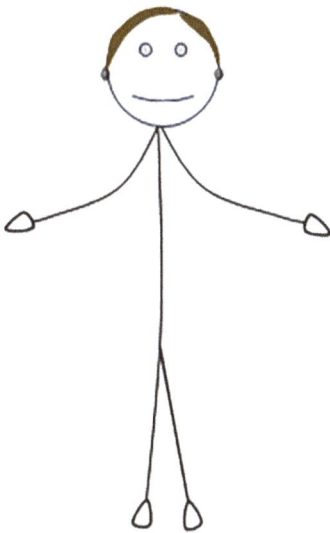
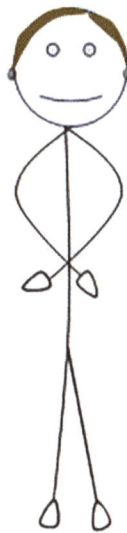
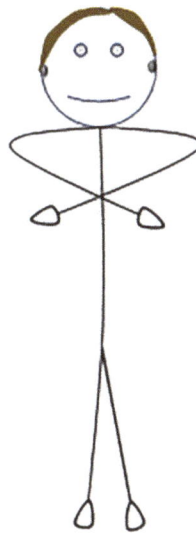
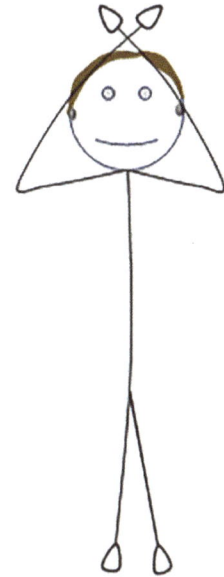

5)

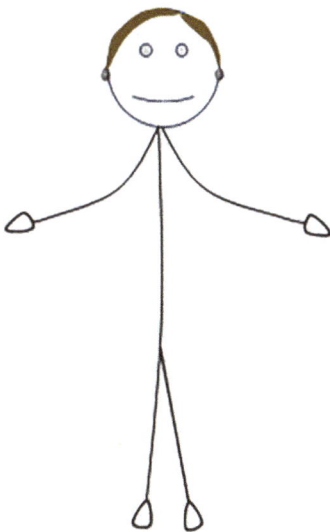

Rotating your arms in an inwards sweep, five times. Then rotate your arms in an outwards sweep five times. As you do the exercise, make sure your sweeping arms cover your body from the lower part to your head. Once done, then back to the beginning, and repeat. Allow your arms to feel loose and almost disconnected to your body, Enjoy the exercise and feel the freedom it brings into your life, and your breathing. Do not overdo the exercise. Once done always give yourself a break of thirty seconds, take a sip of water. The important point of exercising: <u>repeat them on a regular basis.</u>

It's an interesting point, bones grow in our body to allow us to do the daily work or activities to live our daily lives. Muscles are developed in our body to support our bones. Muscles help us to move easily and again, to do the daily activities we need to do, to survive.

As people become older, some, not all, forget about their body muscles and rely on their bones to operate taking over the muscles work. Good health will only decline if we do not keep our muscles healthy through exercise!

SUMMARY OF MODULE ONE

You have learnt:

- ✓ How to understand your different personality states.
- ✓ How having a shower before you exercise, helps with muscle movement and enjoyment of the exercise journey.
- ✓ How to move your arms in a way that helps with breathing, relaxation and the reduction of stress which all contribute to your overall health and wellbeing.

END OF MODULE ONE

MODULE TWO
BREATHING – IT IS THE MOST IMPORTANT PART OF YOUR EXERCISE JOURNEY – HEAD EXERCISES AND WRIST MOVEMENTS

In this module you will learn:

- ✓ How to breathe properly.
- ✓ Talking about your personal esteem.
- ✓ How to do head movements, which help to release your body's stress.
- ✓ How to exercise feet, ankle, and leg muscles, which helps in general physical movements.
- ✓ Caring for your feet and giving them the love, they deserve.

Wanting to know more about how your body works is part of your journey in getting to know about you! The human body and brain are made up of a collection of mainly moving parts, for instance, your heart pumps blood, your lungs help you to breathe; many people know the outcome of having different infections or lung conditions and when these moving parts become sick! We only need to think about the recent Covid pandemic to realise how important the human lungs and good health really are! Likewise, the human brain, though the brain doesn't move like a physical muscle as in an arm or leg, it has electronic parts that move throughout the brain, which relay messages from your brain to other parts of your body. For instance, you want to make a cup of tea, the body cannot take the action, 1) move your legs, 2) go to the kettle, 3) fill it with water, 4) turn on the power to allow the water to boil; none of these actions will happen unless your brain's electronics are working properly! So, as mature adults, we are all responsible for keeping all working parts in good order, and mainly the good order comes from eating a healthy diet, doing the exercises needed to keep the limbs and muscles healthy and being aware that the brain is also a vital part of the human body and its functions.

LET'S TALK ABOUT YOUR PERSONAL ESTEEM...

As we become older, our body needs a lot more love and attention, and it is only us, the owner of the body, that can give that needed attention to ourselves. Part of aging can lead to having a low self-esteem, that low self-esteem can show in the way we hold ourselves within our posture. It is important, as you undergo this new awareness of 'SELF', that you remember to, 1) stand straight, 2) pull your shoulders back, 3) hold your head high, and be proud of who you are.

When I go shopping or walk down the street, I see so many beautiful people, (and there are some people who have health conditions that may make them slump forward), but if you do not, do not allow 'premature slumping' to interfere with your self-esteem, posture, health, and wellbeing.

LET'S LEARN THE ART OF BREATHING

When your breathing is erratic, you will build up more carbon dioxide than your body needs.

A build-up of too much carbon dioxide can add to accumulated stress in your body and make you feel anxious, and nervous, when you possibly have no reason to feel that way...!

I want to say here, there are many experts who know a lot about breathing, but for now, it is time to relax and start the simple breathing journey. Once you are familiar with breathing, then please look for other techniques that may support you in your health and wellbeing.

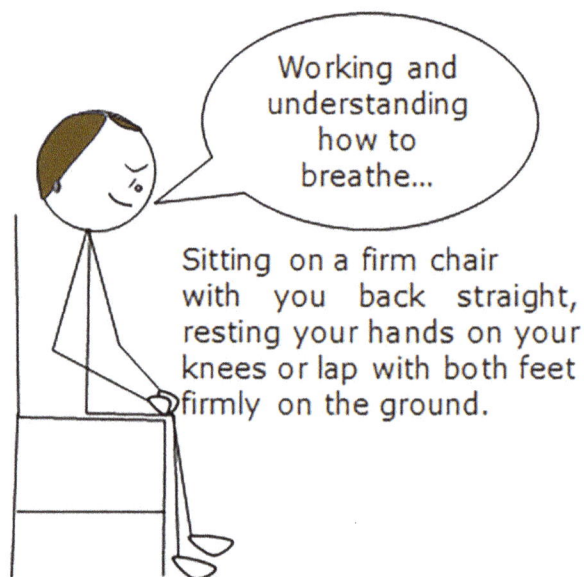

Working and understanding how to breathe...

Sitting on a firm chair with you back straight, resting your hands on your knees or lap with both feet firmly on the ground.

A good time to do breathing exercises is when you are having your shower or bath.

Lift your head high and feel proud of who you are.

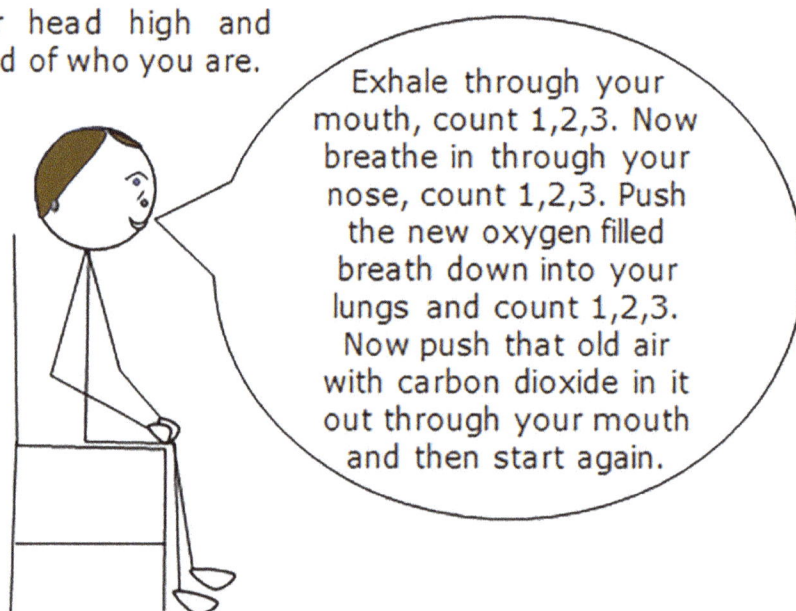

Exhale through your mouth, count 1,2,3. Now breathe in through your nose, count 1,2,3. Push the new oxygen filled breath down into your lungs and count 1,2,3. Now push that old air with carbon dioxide in it out through your mouth and then start again.

Try to keep your back as straight as possible and lift your shoulders high so that you expand your diaphragm.

Do the breathing exercises seen on the previous page, five times. If you can manage ten, then go to ten.

Once the exercises are done, it's now time to take a thirty second break, maybe a sip of water and then we'll start working with your head movements.

Please remember, always, always, keep in mind your breathing as you do your exercises.

SIDE TO SIDE HEAD MOVEMENTS

Moving your head from side to side, count to ten. Do five movements on each side, then rest for thirty seconds.

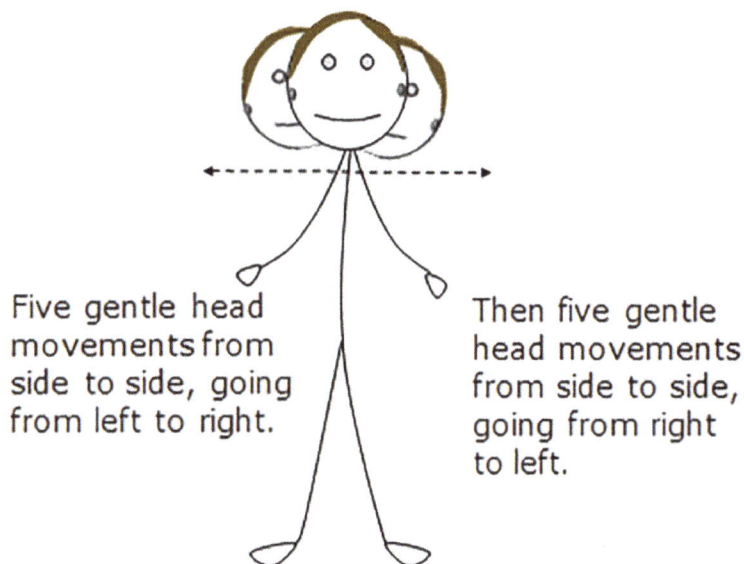

Five gentle head movements from side to side, going from left to right.

Then five gentle head movements from side to side, going from right to left.

Once rested from doing the head movement exercises from side to side, then do the following exercises moving your head forward and back.

FORWARD AND BACK HEAD MOVEMENTS

Standing proud, with your back straight, shoulders back, move your head forward, then back. Do this exercise for five, then rest. How do you feel?

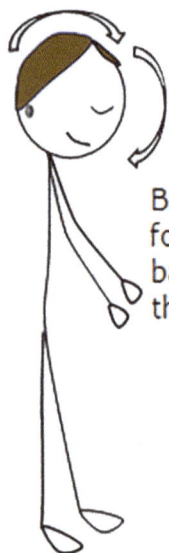

Bring your head forward, then back, forward, then back...

BACK AND FORWARD HEAD MOVMEMENTS

Keeping your head and neck flexible with exercising, improves everyday body movement.

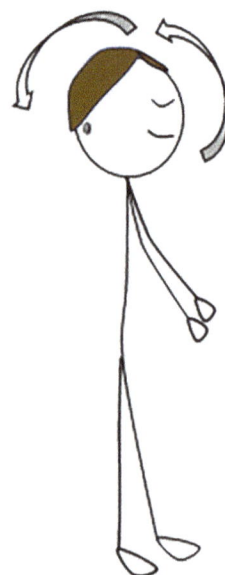

Bring your head back, then forward, then back...

By doing this exercise, you stretch your neck muscles but listen to what your body is telling you. You can only do so much in the beginning. Each time of day you do these exercises, and (please try to do them every second or third day...), you will find that your body becomes so much more flexible.

WRIST MOVEMENTS AND ROTATIONS

As we are exercising our upper body, you will need to think about your arms and wrists. Your hands are important parts of your body, and they too, need to be kept in good order.

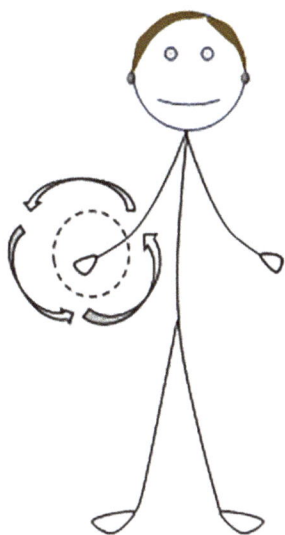

Rotate your hand, which in turn will exercise your wrist, do these five to ten times. Remembering to do the number of turns that feel comfortable for you. Then go in the opposite direction with your same hand and wrist movement. Once you are satisfied with the number of wrist movements, then go to your opposite wrist and repeat the exercise.

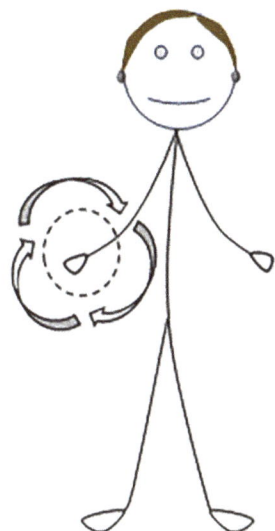

When you have finished this exercise, you have completed module two, so, congratulations, but this is not the end, it is just the beginning of your new life journey.

Now, please take some time out and thank you for committing to your own very good health.

SUMMARY OF MODULE TWO

You have learnt:

- ✓ How to breathe and the techniques of breathing.
- ✓ How to move your head in forward and back movements and working to your own pace and body's capacity.
- ✓ How rotate your wrist and ankles.
- ✓ Learning how to strengthen your feet and legs.

END OF MODULE TWO

MODULE THREE
LET'S TALK ABOUT YOUR BRAIN AND THE FOOD YOU EAT...! EXERCISING YOUR LEGS, ANKLES AND FEET

In this module you will learn:

- ✓ How to look for healthy food without food additive numbers.
- ✓ How to rotate and exercise your ankles in sitting and standing positions.
- ✓ How to keep your feet in good working condition.
- ✓ How to strengthen your leg muscles. and
- ✓ The standup, sit down exercise.

The food and drink we consume is the fuel we put in our human body, our tanks!

When I'm speaking to the students in a classroom, we may discuss food and what is healthy food, what is 'junk food?' and other aspects of the food and drink available on the supermarket shelves.

The question at this point, if you drive an expensive car or a car you care about, you need to ask yourself, 'would I put rubbish fuel in the tank of my car...?' If you put rubbish fuel in your car, your car will, generally, give you rubbish performance...! So, it is wise to treat your car and your body with the respect it deserves, and that means putting the recommended fuel in your car and eating a good, healthy, wholesome diet.

In module two, I spoke about your brain, and now to continue that conversation. Once you acknowledge your brain and become aware, that your brain is a complex organ that works with giving signals that allow you to do the exercise movements you need to do. Your brain is more complexed than any computer developed to date. In exercising, you are giving your brain the commands your body needs to do which allows you, for example, to rotate your head, move your hands in rotation which allows you to exercise your wrists and so on.

Your brain is a remarkable tool, but you need to be in control of how you work with it, and the commands you give it. It is like putting your car into gear, if you want to go forward, would you put the gear into reverse? Of course, you would not! Having said that, many people may work with their brain in reverse because they cannot move forward...!

You give your brain the information in the thoughts you have. Your thoughts show in the actions you take and the words you speak, also, your brain is conditioned by you. The conditioning is brought about by the way you think, experiences you've had and the attitude you develop! The brain is a tool, and the way we use this tool is, in most instances, up to us.

On this journey, you are making new changes to your thinking and behaviour. You are now wanting a new direction to your own health and wellbeing. This book, the words and illustrations are about your new beginning and the positive changes you are making.

With new thinking a behaviour, you will see the world differently. You will see new opportunities, talk with new people who may have similar interests to you; you can, in many instances, change the way you live in the world.

With new and positive changes made, you will find a new and different awareness to you as an individual and human being.

Learning to exercise your body is developing your motor skills. Motor skills are a combination of life skills you have learnt during your life. You need all your skills to work during exercising and living from this day and forward into the future.

Your brain, as I have said, controls your thoughts, it also controls your memory, breathing, emotion, and your body's temperature. It also regulates your senses, which include hearing, seeing, touching, smelling, and tasting. Together with the above, it also powers your hunger states which allows messages to go from your gut, through your spinal cord, then to your brain. Your brain continually interacts with all parts of your body which is connected to your central nervous system, your (CNS).

In the last paragraph, I have mentioned your hunger states, and this brings me to the quality of the food you eat. When exercising, you need to eat, good, whole, unadulterated food; this means your food needs to be from naturally grown sources and cooked without harmful food additives.

I have been a writer of many books, and one book took over five years to research, write and publish, that book is 'Devils In Our Food'.

The findings within the research for this book were frightening.

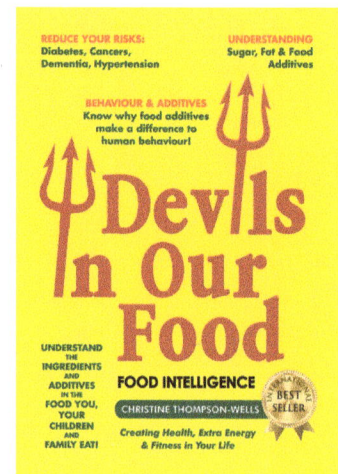

When I first started the research into food additives, I found about three-hundred and twenty additives mentioned on the Australian Government website. Seven years later, our latest research reveals there are up to or more than ten thousand food additives going into the manufactured and processed world food supply chain.

The research revealed, that out of all manufactured foods, flour had the greatest number of 'dangerous' food additives. There are many additives going into a range of breads, cakes, biscuits, and those foods that have flour included as part of their ingredients.

I have copied some of the additives, their related numbers, and names from my book, seen in the above. Seeing these, it may remind you to look on the ingredients panel on the food labels next time you go food shopping.

Out of over forty dangerous additives going into flour and everyday food products, I am showing you just a few on these pages.

150d **Avoid**	Caramel IV Ammonia sulphite process
Colour: Rich dark brown Known as 4-Mel is a sulfite ammonia. Acid-proof caramel used in many drink and food products. Stable in alcohol, tannin, and acid-rich environments. Used in soft and fizzy drinks and other carbonated beverages, balsamic vinegar, coffee, chocolate syrups, baked goods, cocoa extenders, pet food, sauces, soy sauce, soups, meat rubs, seasoning blends, beer, biscuits, cakes, chocolate, confectionary, sweets and lollies, crisps, doughnuts, flour products, fruit sauces, ice cream, pickles, oyster sauce, pâté, preserves, soy sauce, whiskey, wine, meat, and vegetable substitutes. Is known to cause asthma, hyperactivity, hypersensitivity, gastrointestinal disorder, and liver problems. Carbohydrates and ammonia are used to produce caramel. The Centre for Science in the Public Interest (CSPI**)**. *'… the FDA immediately should change the name 'caramel colouring' to 'chemically modified caramel colouring' or 'ammonia-sulfite process caramel colouring' and should not allow products to be labelled 'natural' if they contain any type of caramel colouring.'*[1] Is linked to asthma, hyperactivity, hypersensitivity, gastrointestinal conditions, liver problems. Also linked to: *'birth defects, neurological disorders, negative effects on the immune system, decrease in white blood cells, convulsions.'*[2] See 150b. Also causes vitamin B deficiency. Approved in the United States, European Union, New Zealand, and Australia. **Avoid**

---

[1] http://www.befoodsmart.com Source: Centre for Science in the Public Interest.
[2] http://thearticlebay.com

173 **Avoid**	Aluminium

Colour: silver grey

There is no dietary requirement within the human body for this additive. Is used in sugar-coated and flour confectionary decorations and in the presentation of dragées (small bite-sized confectionary with a hard, external shell). May be used in other foods and drinks. Is linked to premature senility, Parkinson's and Alzheimer's disease, osteoporosis, some kidney disease, toxicity of the nervous system, cardiovascular system, the reproductive and respiratory systems. Banned in some countries. On alert in the United States. Approved in the European Union, New Zealand, and Australia. **Avoid**

220 **Avoid**	Sulphur dioxide

Colour: A strong pungent gas

A preservative obtained from coal tar. Is produced by the combustion of sulphur and gypsum. In the United States, the use of this product is prohibited on fresh fruit and vegetables. Used in wine making and for preservation of dried prunes, apricots, raisins, and dried fruits. Found in beer, juices, cordials, vinegar, and prepared potato products. Used as a bleaching agent in flour. Reduces absorption of vitamin B1 and other B vitamins. May cause wheezing in asthmatics, difficulty in breathing if you aren't asthmatic, facial swelling or hive type skin reactions. Is difficult to metabolize for people with impaired kidney function. Is linked to: *'birth defects, genetic damage, nerve damage, behavioural disorders in children, unconsciousness, seizures, swelling in the brain, vomiting, visual disturbance, and severe allergic reactions. Approximately 30-40 people die each year in the United States because of 220 – 228.'*[3] Not recommended for babies or young children. Approved in the United States, European Union, New Zealand, and Australia. **Avoid**

---

[3] http://thearticlebay.com

221 Avoid	Sodium sulphite, sulfite

Colour: White powder with a faint odour of sulphur dioxide

Is a sulphite decontaminating agent used in fresh orange juice. Sulphites are added to many fruit drinks, sausages, dried fruits, fresh fruits and vegetables, beer, wine, fruit juices, sauces, frozen shellfish, bread, egg yolk products, caramel, salads, and other foods. They destroy vitamin B1, B12 and vitamin E. Used to protect food and beverages from microorganisms and oxidation. May cause severe reactions in asthmatics, cause headaches, migraine, intestinal upset, skin disorders and ailments, eczema, and dermatitis; creates behavioural problems, can contribute to ADHD, cause gastric irritation and nausea. Approved in the United States, European Union, New Zealand and Australia. **Avoid**

223 Avoid	Sodium metabisulphate

Colour: White crystals or crystalline powder – has an odour of sulphur dioxide

Is used as a flour bleaching agent, preservative, disinfectant, and antioxidant. Is used in beer and wine making. Also used in sausages, dried raisins, dates, apples, frozen vegetables, vinegar, apple cider vinegar, fruit concentrate juices, concentrated tomato juice, cereal, muesli, cracker biscuits, paste, pulp, puree, canned vegetables and fruits, frozen French fries, fruit syrups, fruit fillings, marmalade, jellies, sugar syrups, pickled condiments, coleslaw, sauerkraut, mustard, relish, ketchup, soy products, (tofu), snack foods, dried spices, herbs, tea, processed potatoes, shell and fish products, fresh grapes, glazed and glace fruits. Not recommended for children. Can cause respiratory reactions in asthmatics. May cause gastric irritation and intestinal discomfort. Contributes to nettle rash, swelling and skin reactions including: eczema, dermatitis, itching, hives and rashes. Can cause behavioural problems; contribute to ADHD and difficulties in learning. May cause headaches and migraine. Approved in the United States, European Union, New Zealand and Australia. **Avoid**

406 **Avoid**	Agar or agar agar

Colour: White and semi-translucent powder
Is a nonorganic, non-synthetic vegetable gum derived from red seaweed. Is a soluble fibre and additive used in pie fillings, meringues, glazing, cream, milk, yogurt, meringue shells, sherbets, ice cream, canned and cured manufactured meats, noodles, cheeses, sauces, baked products, cakes, icings, jelly, candies, sweets, confectionary, fondants, and many Asian desserts. Can cause flatulence and distension in the abdomen. *'Is linked to cancer.'*[4] Agar, agar approved in the United States, European Union, New Zealand, and Australia. **Avoid**

Some of the numbers and names in the above may alarm you, but all that is needed is vigilance and asking the food conglomerates three detailed questions:

1. How is this food or drink produced?
2. What are the ingredients in this food or drink?
3. Is this food or drink good for me to swallow and for my health?

You may wish to do some of your own research into the food you buy, there are many websites you can scroll.

NOW, BACK TO EXERCISING

We finalised the last module with doing wrist and hand rotation exercises. To extend your movements, let's now move to your ankles and feet.

---

[4] http://thearticlebay.com

EXERCISING YOUR ANKLES AND FEET

If you haven't exercised for a long time, you may like to stay sitting on your chair, but to gain balance or to start to re-align your body's weight and balance, you may wish to stand for the next ankle and leg exercises.

With a sturdy and firm table or chair in your visual sight we will begin.

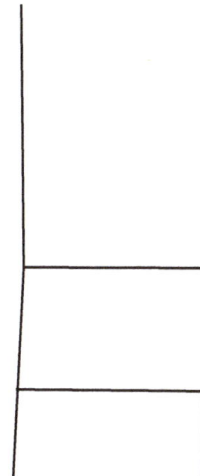

Stand if you can. Standing can help to re-align your body weight.

As I have said, make sure you have a firm and stable surface or a surface that is fixed; having this visual and sturdy base within reach while exercising will help you to maintain balance.

STANDING ON ONE LEG, COUNT TO TEN

Make sure you feel secure, and you have control of your balance with your hand supporting you. As seen in the illustration, you may wish to use a nearby table or chair for this support.

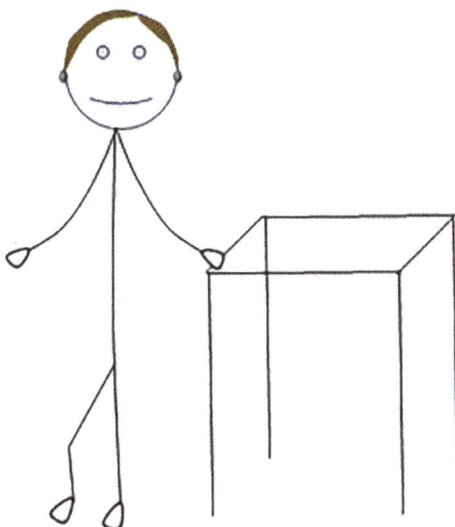

Gaining the sense of strength back into your body is always a good start to gaining good, positive health and making the most of what you have. Now, count to ten.

Do the same with the opposite leg, if needed, keep yourself secure by supporting your body with your hand resting on the secure base. On one leg, stand still, and count to ten.

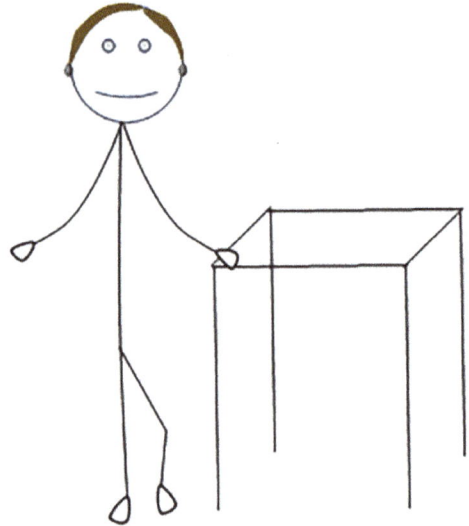

ROTATING YOUR FOOT – LEFT THEN RIGHT

Rotate your foot, thus moving your ankle to the right five to ten times. Then rotate in the opposite direction for five to ten times. Stop, relax and then we'll start on the left foot. Use which ankle feels the most comfortable to start with.

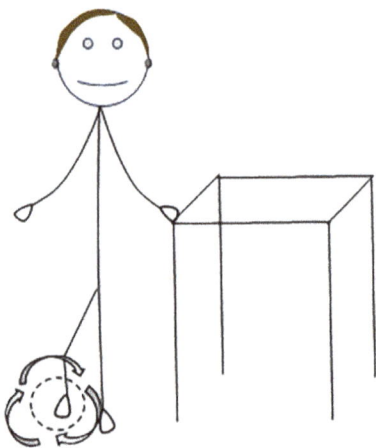

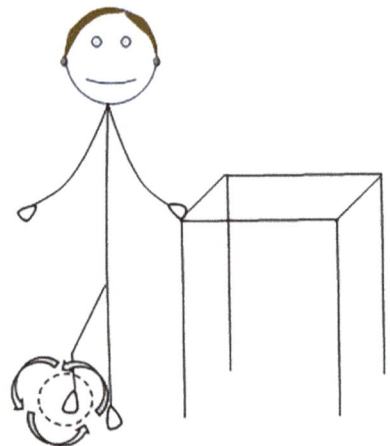

By rotating your ankle, with the guidance from your big toe, you can go either clockwise, then anticlockwise.

Once you have rotated your foot going in your chosen direction, then change and go in the opposite direction.

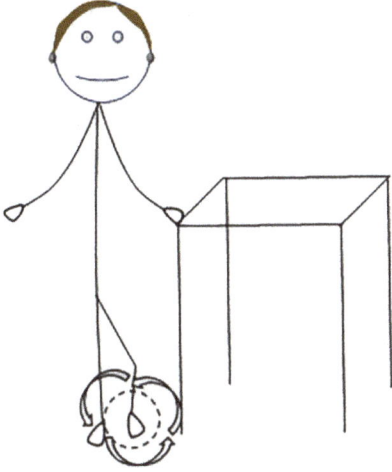

Now going to the opposite leg, rotating your foot five to ten times going clockwise, then anticlockwise.

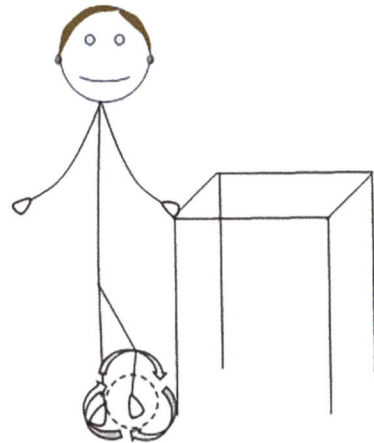

Always keep your exercising actions even. Remember, continue to do the same number of movements going in both directions.

A part of the body that is often missed in exercising, are our feet. If your feet are neglected, they will let you know by becoming tired, they may also show displeasure with broken skin and skin breakouts that make it difficult for you to walk and to enjoy everyday life and activities.

MOVING YOUR TOES IN THE DIRECTION OF YOUR KNEE

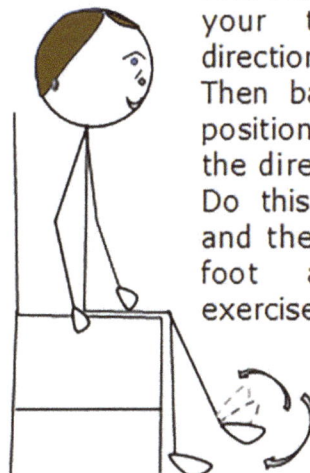

Sitting back on the chair and while your ankles and feet are limbered up, bring your toes up in the direction of the knee.
Then back to the original position, then back up into the direction of your knee. Do this five to ten times and then go to your other foot and repeat the exercise.

Our feet are a marvellous human part of our anatomy. They go with us everywhere; they take us on many journeys throughout life, and as we become older, they need a little bit more consideration...!

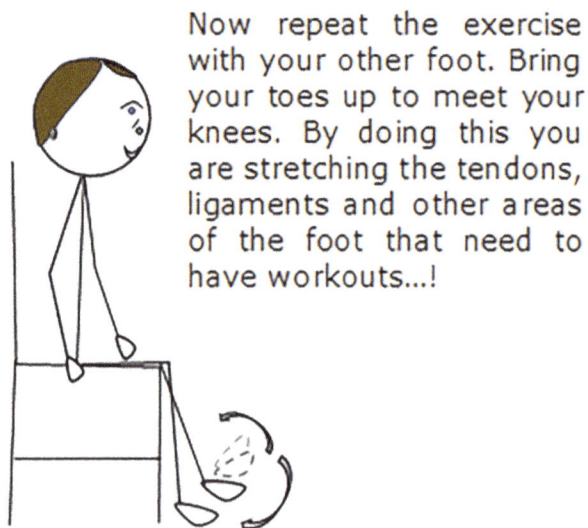

Now repeat the exercise with your other foot. Bring your toes up to meet your knees. By doing this you are stretching the tendons, ligaments and other areas of the foot that need to have workouts...!

By doing regular foot and ankle exercises, the blood flows freely, the ligaments, muscles, and other connecting and supporting foot parts stay in good condition, and this good work supports you as you continue your life journey.

STRENGTHENING YOUR LEGS

Now, let's go to your legs, legs need to be worked, working legs are essential to good health. Regardless of how you feel each day, you need to use your legs through walking, exercising, dancing or a definite exercise that helps the wellbeing of your legs. I have seen unused legs, and it is sad, leg muscles seem to almost 'slip away' when they are not used. Everyday leg muscles must be put into action and used every day!

STENGTHENING YOUR ANKLES AND LEGS

There are many ways to keep your body healthy, it does take time, but it is well worth the investment for your long-term health.

Sitting on your chair, secure an exercise stretchable or sizable elastic band firmly to either the leg of a bed or onto a firmly fixed base. Secure your foot into the band, pulling your foot in and out by stretching.

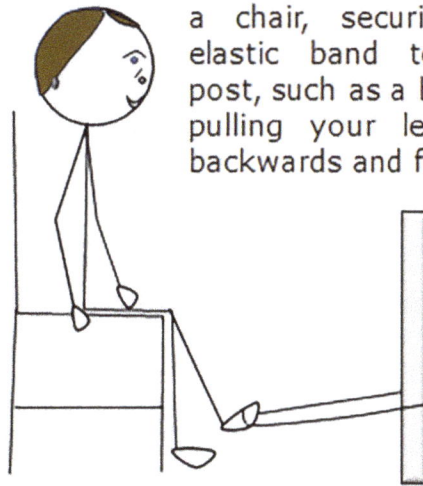

Other ways of strengthening your feet and ankle muscles can be done while sitting on a chair, securing a large elastic band to a secure post, such as a bed post and pulling your leg and foot backwards and forwards.

During all exercises try to remember your breathing. Now move your foot backwards and forward or 'in and out', and listen to your breathing, follow the rhythm so that your leg exercises correspond with your breathing pattern. Do the exercises for five to ten times on one foot, then change to the other foot.

STRENGHTHENING YOUR FEET

In the opposite illustration, you can see how the right toes on the right leg are bent forward. Your body weight is supported by your opposite leg and foot which stays firmly on the ground.

Exercising the bottom of your foot is equally as important as exercising other areas of your feet and body.

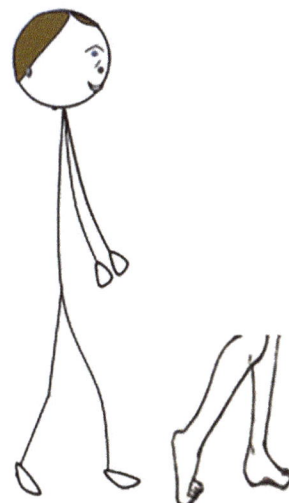

Now repeat this exercise on your opposite foot. Bending

your toes forward by using your body's strength helps in building foot strength. This exercise also helps in aligning your body's balance, strengthening your leg, ancle, and foot muscles, while strengthening your foot tendons and the moving parts of your foot.

This exercise is not only good for your under-foot muscles, but also the areas of the fasciitis ligament, and calf muscles.

When your feet are exercised, and as a bonus to yourself, at the end of this session, and after the exercises, sit down, make a cup of tea, and with some moisturiser, give your feet a well-earned massage. Once massaged, let the ointment do its work, but remove any excess, give your feet a light rinse with warm water, and towel dry. Do not walk anywhere with wet feet.

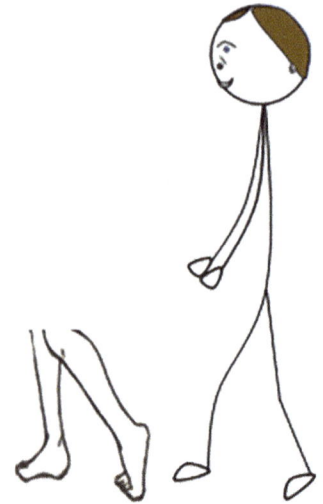

By giving your feet this quality time, you will be amazed at how you feel. The time spent is completely worth the investment made.

PAYING MORE ATTENTION TO YOUR LEGS – SIDEWAYS MOVEMENTS – SWEEPING YOUR LEG OUT AND BACK

As I have previously said, 'Our legs carry us through life,' and sometimes our legs and body feel tired, and they don't want to work! It is precisely at these times when we must make our legs and body work. Giving in to the brain sending you a negative message of 'I can't exercise today, I'm just too tired...!' is not an option. If you have set your goals yesterday to do your exercises today, doing your exercises you must do – it is clearly as simple as that.

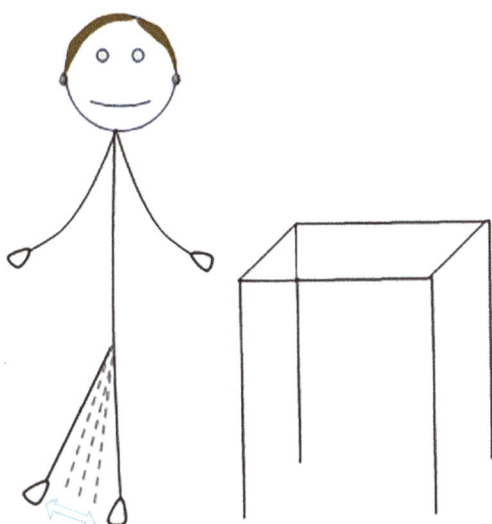

Keeping your table or secure base in sight, you are ready to start this new leg exercise. Please remember, you are the driver in the control seat of your vehicle, your body is your vehicle and sometimes, your brain and body become stubborn...!

As you do this exercise, move your leg out sideways as far as you can reach; you may start with small sideway movements, and then move your leg out and up further as you gain confidence in what you are doing.

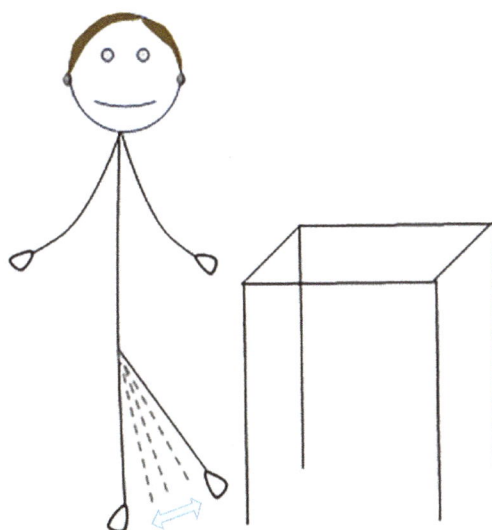

If you do have days when exercising seems 'just too hard,' think of the benefits and wellbeing you feel after the time spent on you, and this thinking will change your attitude that allows you to continue with your exercises.

USING YOUR LEGS TO THEIR MAXIMUM ADVANTAGE – STAND UP – SIT DOWN

Stand in front of a chair and face a secure table or bar to secure yourself if you need support. A bar or strong table will help you to keep your balance as you become familiar with this new exercise. Place the chair behind you but in front of the firm table or something strong you can hold on to until you find your confidence and balance. Facing the table, we will begin.

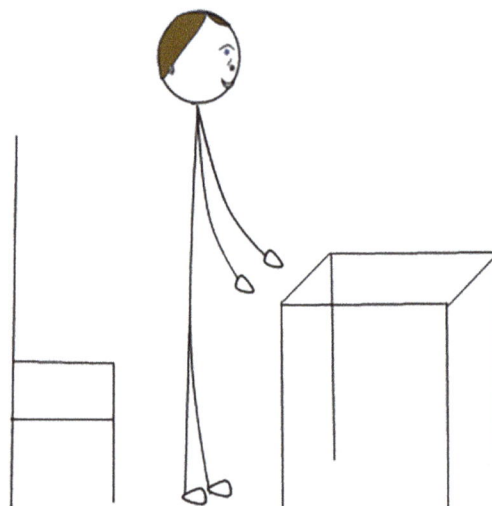

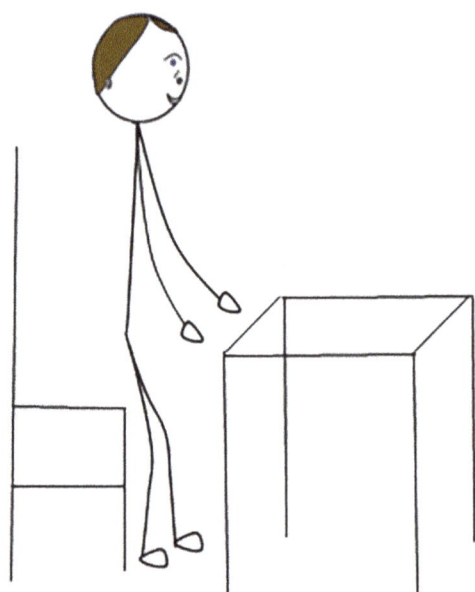

The chair is not for you to sit on, but as a support if you think you are losing your balance as you stretch and grow with confidence while doing this exercise.

With your feet firmly on the ground, remembering your breathing:

1) Breathe out through your mouth and count to three as you start to lower your body.

(Please remember, you are not in a race or competing with anybody else, so please take this exercise slowly.)

2) Holding your breath, count to three, bend your knees to a level you feel comfortable with. As you come back to fully standing, with your back straight and your legs fully upright,

3) Let the old breath out.

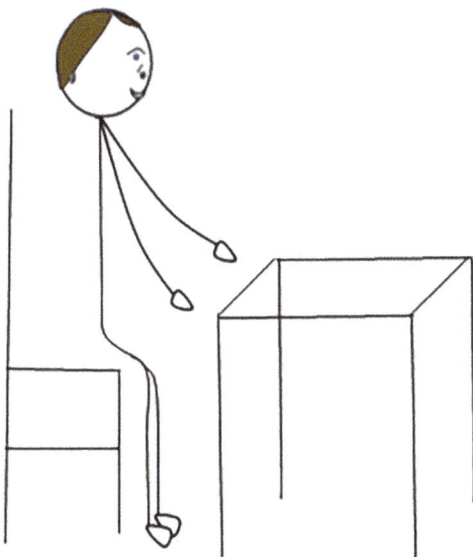

As we become older, because of the lack of use of our limbs, we slowly lose confidence in what we so easily did when we were younger. If you are in good general health, your muscles will still want to work for you.

By extending and stretching yourself to go just a little bit further each day, you will soon have your vitality and energy levels back. You may even surprise yourself in just how good you feel!

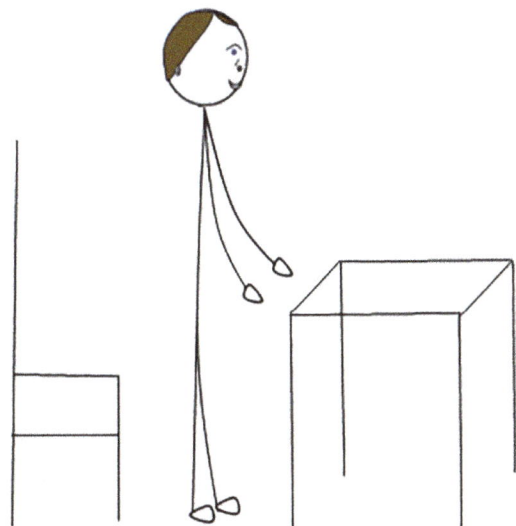

SUMMARY OF MODULE THREE

You have learnt:

- ✓ How important eating healthy food is to maintain a healthy body.
- ✓ How to rotate and exercise your arms, ankles, and legs.
- ✓ How important it is to keep your feet and legs in good working order and condition.
- ✓ The standup, sit down exercise.

END OF MODULE THREE

MODULE FOUR
THE MOLECULES IN YOUR FOOD AND DRINK – KNEE LIFTS AND MORE LEG EXERCISES

In this module you will learn:

- ✓ Knowing more about food additives and how food molecules are changed from natural to manipulated molecules.
- ✓ Knowing more about how the Quadricep (quad) and Gluteal (glute) knee muscles work.
- ✓ How to effectively work with your knees, and
- ✓ How to keep your knees healthy.

FIRST, BACK TO TEACHING

Teaching children and young people has many great rewards, from the expression on their faces when they learn something new, to their eagerness of wanting to know more about the new information they have just been taught.

At one of my sessions with a class of over thirty, extremely bright students at a local school, I ventured into the food debate, though food was mentioned in the information I was given to teach, it was very light and without any real substance to the 'HOW?' and 'WHY?' food information debate I was trying to bring into the lesson information.

LET'S GET BACK TO THE FOOD DEBATE

So, what is a molecule? Molecules are all around us, they are in the water we drink, the food we eat, the air we breathe, and we, within our bodies, are indeed made up of a collection of molecules. The human body, though we are living in the 21st Century, is an ancient system and never in human history, has the human body been so invaded by synthetic and manipulated molecules in the food we eat and the drinks we drink as in our lifetime in this century.

So, what is a molecule? Each molecule is small, so small, they can only be seen under a microscope. In a simple explanation, each molecule is made up of 1) a fatty head, 2) has three legs and, 3) is a combination of hydrogen and carbon chains within the legs.

In a simple explanation, the chains of the molecule can vary in length, and this is all to do with where the molecule has come from. Is it from protein as in meat, fish, or another source of protein? These are all complicated questions which science has answered over many years of food science research. Protein and carbohydrate have different lengths in the chemical chain of the molecule.

To satisfy the market demand for longer lasting, or longer 'shelf life' foods, tasty, colourful, and easy to make foods, food developers have worked with trans fats that are used in the

46

everyday, manufactured and processed worldwide food chain. Trans fats are fats that have had their carbon chains modified to meet the food demand for longer lasting, cookie-cut looking, manufactured cheap and fast foods, but trans fats are also used in many well-known brand products bought by families worldwide.

MOVING THE MOLECULE

Briefly, Trans-fat is a manmade product first developed in 1809 by Paul Sabatier a Nobel prize winner for his work in Chemistry. In 1901, Wilhelm Normann, a German chemist showed that liquid oils could be hydrogenated and patented the process in 1902. Normann's process of hydrogenation showed that whale and fish oil could be stabilised and used for human consumption.

From that time and onwards, trans fats have been used in margarines, cooking oils, manufactured foods, and other commercial food products.

YOUR BODY ENZYMES Vs ALTERED AND MODIFIED MOLECULES OF THE 21ST CENTURY

Herein, lies the problems to many of the current day health conditions and sickness.

Again, the human system is an ancient system and the enzymes within your body have been handed down from many of your ancestors over many thousands of years. The molecules in many of today's food products are new and altered molecules. These altered molecules are not recognised by the enzymes in your intestines, stomach, pancreas, and saliva.

Your natural body's enzymes breakdown fats, proteins, and carbohydrates. They help in your breathing, building body muscle, ridding your body of dangerous toxins and in cell repair. When food containing altered molecules is eaten, these natural enzymes cannot do their work; therefore, the altered molecules stay in your body. They are unable to go through the natural process of being expelled from your body by the faeces released.

If your food, is natural and from uncontaminated sources, the natural molecules are left in place and your natural body enzymes can do their work in keeping you healthy.

When natural foods are eaten, your body can do the body repairs it needs to do when damage occurs, and as we become older, many of us suffer from damaged joints, and the knees are no exception to painful damage.

STRENGTHENING YOUR KNEE JOINTS AND THE MUSCLES AROUND YOUR KNEES

Most of us know the discomfort of pain if a knee or both knees are not working properly! In many instances painful knee joints can be brought on through lack of exercise, or not understanding how our knees work!

I too, have damage a knee through wearing the wrong shoes and walking too far in those wrong shoes! It took about ten years, from one night out, for my knee to repair. Love, tender care and thinking about the shoes I will wear for different occasions are now a priority in my thinking when going out or to some special event!

I have mentioned working with a personal trainer before and while I write this book. I have learnt a lot about my legs and their importance in keeping my legs, especially my knees in good working condition. I now understand the words: quadriceps and gluteal muscles and their importance in keeping our knees, legs, and lower body healthy, and how these muscles and their work need to be understood.

1. Quadriceps, (quads): are the muscles that run along the side of the leg and connect to the knee. These muscles support the knee to keep straight to absorb shock when doing activities like walking, running, exercising and other weight-bearing activities or jobs! If, for instance, like me, you wear the wrong shoes, then this, or these muscles can be damaged!

2. Gluteal (glutes): are the muscles that support the hip and leg muscles, (both your hips and legs have the ability to rotate inwards or outwards), this movement can only be done through the help of your glute muscles. Because most of us sit in a chair, far more than our ancestors have ever

done, our glutes become weak and, in some instances, almost unworkable!

3. There are three main parts to the gluteal muscle, they work with your buttocks, and stretch from your back hipbone to the top of your thigh bone. They are 1, gluteus maxims, 2, gluteus medius, and 3, gluteus minimus. These muscles help you to stabilise your lower limbs, including the pelvis.

From this point on, you are now ready to get your knees into good working order.

RAISING YOUR KNEES

If you haven't done any leg exercises for some time, you may wish to sit on a firm sofa or dining room chair to do this knee exercise!

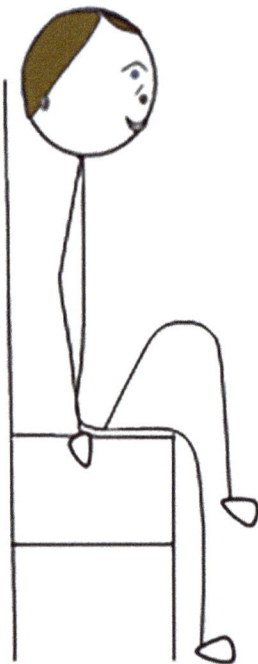

First, raise your leg, bending your knee and lift it as high as possible keeping your lower leg and foot firmly on the floor, and as straight as you can. Hold the raised knee position, and count to five, if you can manage ten, then stretch yourself and do the extra counts.

Once you are happy with your first effort, then exercise the other leg in the same way. When you have met your goal, try, and do this exercise daily or every second day, and you will be amazed at the energy and easier movements that come into your legs.

Keeping in mind, you are working on raising your knees, let's keep the body movements going, let's now move to the 'tummy in, backside out, legs slightly apart' exercise.

TUMMY IN, BACKSIDE OUT, LEGS SLIGHTLY APART

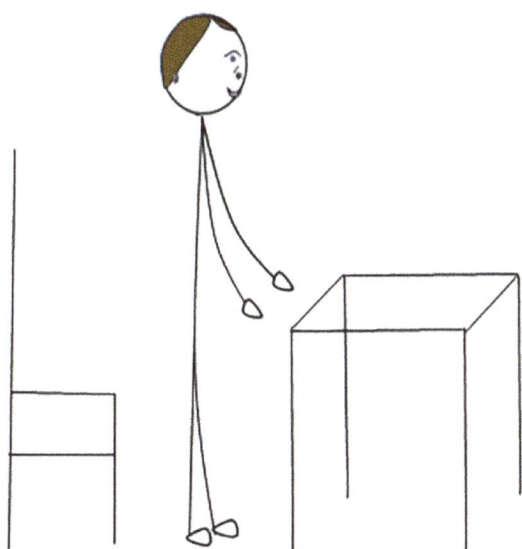

When you are in the position with your secure bench or table in front of you, think of the position your body is in when you are going to sit on a chair! The difference here, your chair is only behind you as your guide, you are not going to sit on it, just use it as a visual and mental tool to keep you safe while you start and go through this exercise. With your feet straight and your legs slightly apart, pull your tummy and their muscles in, force your backside out, bend your knees as though you are about to sit on the chair; go down on your legs as low as you can. Now, lift your body up from your

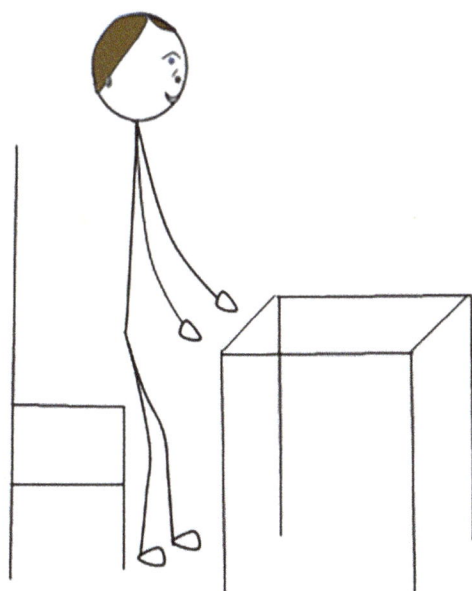

legs and with the help of the strength in your knees, then stand straight.

The more of these bending exercises you do, the stronger your legs and knees will become. Do the tummy in, backside out, legs slightly apart exercise again. Then try to do it at least another three times making it five exercises altogether.

Remember, you are not sitting on the chair, it is only your guide and there to keep you safe!

LEARNING TO SQUAT AGAIN...!

Now, once your confidence is built, keeping the chair in place but away from the table, take the exercise to the next level.

This time, arms outstretched, tummy in, backside out, legs slightly apart, and feet straight, bend your knees and lower your upper body as low as possible, hold that position and count to five, or hold for as long as possible, then stand up straight!

TO BEGIN THE SQUAT - STAND UP STRAIGHT

With your arms outstretched, feet slightly apart, you are ready. Tummy in, backside out, you are ready to put your weight onto your legs and bend your knees.

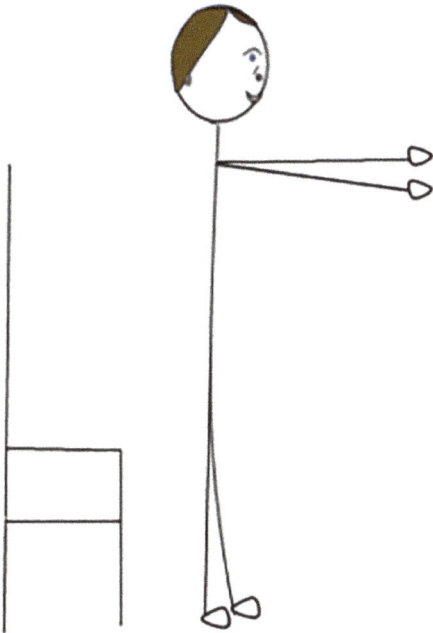

Lower your body down allowing your upper legs and knees to take your weight. Using your legs to support you, go down as far as you can. Once you have achieved your goal, try to count to five, then lift and stand up straight.

In making a target or goal to count to five, you can aim for this with every new squat that you do.

As your body becomes stronger, you will find that you can lower yourself lower and lower each time you attempt to squat. It really is a feeling of accomplishment once you reach your target.

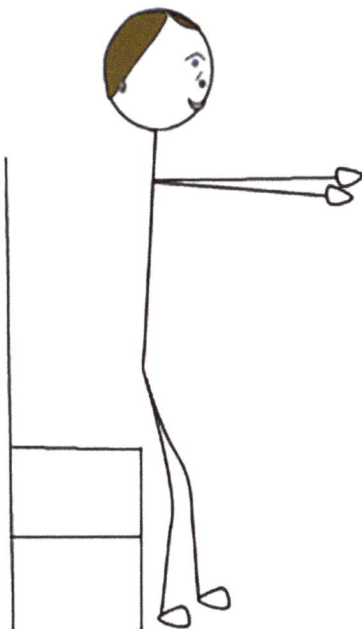

I've just mentioned 'target,' each time you do you're your exercises, aim a little higher; this is your time, and you deserve to get as much out of your effort as possible and recording your achievements is one good way to keep you on track.

By lowering your body down a little lower each time, you do the exercise, you will gain the confidence to continue with your leg strengthening exercises.

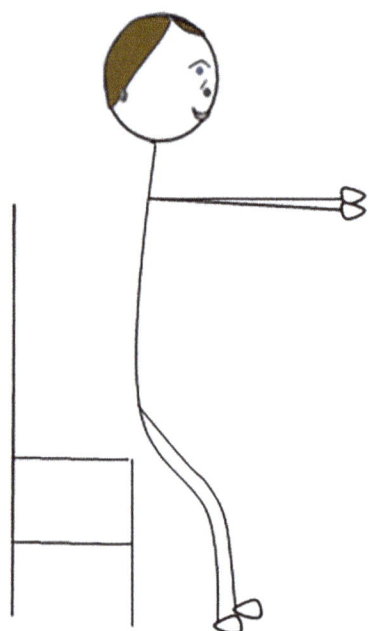

Remembering, you are in control of how you focus and do your exercises, and one way of achieving your goals or targets is to go back time and time again.

Once you achieve your, 'almost sitting' position above the chair, it is time to standup straight and give yourself an 'almighty pat on the back' for achievement.

The feeling of accomplishment as you achieve these major goals will change you and how you see your life.

Many older people want to join groups to do exercises but for some reason, they never seem to 'get around to doing it!' However, by using this book to 'get yourself moving' again, you will see and feel the difference in your self-esteem, confidence, and what you can achieve.

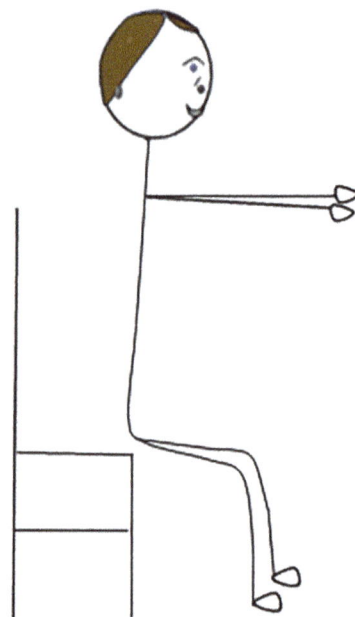

You may wish to do the exercises alone to begin with, but please don't leave your accomplishments in the dark. Tell your friends, family members and those people who may be interested in what you are doing. It is amazing how many people may want to join you on your incredible journey to good health and wellbeing.

WALL SQUATS

This exercise is only done when you feel the confidence to take the next step forward.

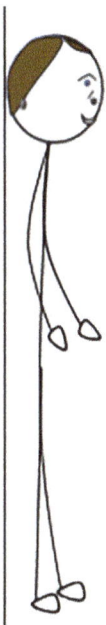

Standing against a wall, making sure the back of your head is touching the wall, keeping your back straight, as you bend your knees, go down as far as you feel comfortable.

The wall will act as a support for your body, but remember, you are in the early stages of getting your body moving and back to good health.

BENDING YOUR KNEES AND LOWERING YOUR BODY – WALL SQUATS

If you want to try new exercises, it is always best to do them with someone else in the room.

By using the wall as your support, bend your knees and lower your body; feel the weight in your legs and how your knees are becoming stronger.

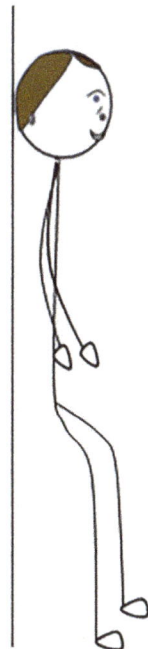

Only go down as far as you feel comfortable. You may find that you only lower yourself a little way, that is fine. The effort of standing straight against a wall, is in itself a very good exercise for strengthening your back muscles.

THE BENEFITS OF KEEPING ACTIVE

✓ By doing exercises, you feel happier.

✓ It helps with keeping your weight down and it becomes easier to lose weight.

✓ Exercise helps with your food digestion and supports your body in its everyday body functions.

✓ Exercise helps with keeping your muscles and bones healthy. You do need to have a daily intake of protein; more about this in Module Five.

✓ Exercise can increase your energy levels.

✓ Exercise can reduce the risk of some chronic diseases, such as diabetes type 2, (exercise adds to your sugar level or glycaemic control), heart disease, many types of cancer, high cholesterol, and other health conditions.

SUMMARY OF MODULE FOUR

You have learnt:

- ✓ About food additives and how food molecules are changed from natural to manipulated molecules.
- ✓ About how the Quadricep (quad) and Gluteal (glute) knee muscles work.
- ✓ How to effectively work with your knees, and
- ✓ How to keep your knees healthy.

END OF MODULE FOUR

MODULE FIVE
THE BENEFITS OF HAVING PURE GELATINE AND MARROW BONE IN THE HUMAN DIET – USING YOUR QUADS TO BETTER HEALTH - GLUTE BRIDGING AND STRENGTHENING YOUR LOWER BODY

In this module you will learn:

- ✓ The benefits of the knowledge from eating naturally grown foods and the advantages of understanding how marrowbone and gelatine support and promote gut and digestive health.
- ✓ How gelatine and marrowbone assist with muscle recovery after exercise or injury; helps to develop strong bones, reduce pain and inflammation in joints and other health benefits.
- ✓ When ready, do the leg raising exercise.
- ✓ When ready, do the glute raising exercise.

It's not much fun, when you want to lie on the floor, but when your legs and knees are not well, they can restrict many natural movements that you took for granted in your younger days!

You are now in the position to make changes to the way your body works; even with some uncomfortable health conditions, with some love, care and work, the body does not become, almost the cage, you are living in but the friend that wants to help you, not only feel better but add to the enjoyment of your everyday life.

Before we get onto the next part of your exercises, I want to speak about the book I've mentioned earlier. The book, Devils In Our Food was a mighty undertaking, and took many thousands of hours to research, write and organise into an easily understood book, that all people could relate to.

Now, many doctors have also found the book helpful and in raising their awareness about food additives, one said to me, 'OK, you've told me all of this information, but what then can I eat?' That question led me on to write a recipe book, entitled, Devil Free Recipes as the cover is seen in the image opposite.

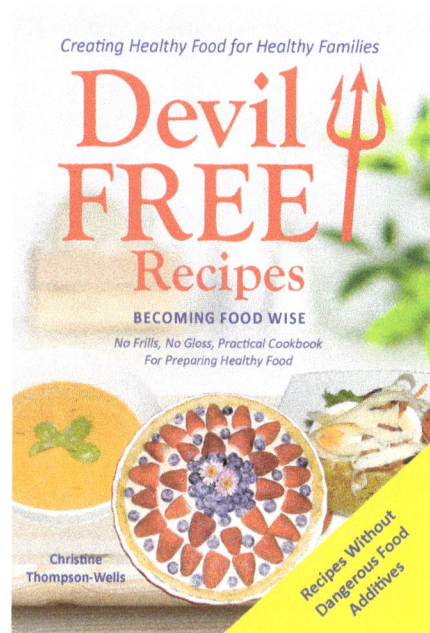

As the year went by, and through the hundreds of recipes I created to produce the book; I didn't want to use any bleached sugar or sugar extracts as an ingredient and did my research into honey and stevia, which are the only two sweeteners I use, but I also wanted to look at food gelling agents. These foods included many desserts, several recipes for children's food, all of which, I wanted to include in the writing and recipes.

As my research continued, and my selection of foods varied, the one miracle ingredient I came across was natural gelatine; it is truly a remarkable ingredient and should be used, instead of synthetic gelling agents, in many foods worldwide! As my research continued, I too, decided to try out exactly how good gelatine really was, the outcome was remarkable.

Though, because of a previous accident with my neck, I have always done some form of regular exercise; the exercise didn't stop the aching groin I had. It was a bit difficult getting in and out of my car, and I could feel the twinge of pain when wanting to climb stairs and do other simple tasks. As I worked on creating the recipes for the book, I eventually got to the dessert section and started reading up on natural gelatine.

When our older generations grew up, fast food was not an option, for the most part, they had good, wholesome cooked foods. Many of the foods included stews, casseroles, and other, basically boiled or oven-cooked food. Often used to flavour soups and stews, were the bones from a previously cooked roast dinner of maybe, beef, lamb, or other roast meat. From the bones, both marrowbone and natural gelatine would leach out into the cooking vegetables and added to the rich flavours of the food.

Marrowbone is not gelatine, but there are similar health benefits from both. In home cooked stews and casseroles, eaten by previous generations, the body would gain the natural, nutritional, goodness of bone broth and gelatine. In the 21st century and with so much manufactured food being consumed, the natural ingredients of foods containing marrowbone and natural gelatine are no longer a part of the everyday diet. This is not good for the world populations and will show in human illness, and severe health conditions in the future.

Bone broth ingredients improve bone health, relieve joint pain, support gut and bowel health and improves your skin. Gelatine is a natural part of the mammal (humans and farmed animals). Unlike marrowbone, which comes from the inside of the bones of animals, gelatine is found in the connective tissue in both bones and joints in farmed animals. The connective tissue includes bones, cartilage, tendons, ligaments, and the skin of animals, it is dried and sold in powder form as collagen and gelatine. Gelatine has a combination of amino acids, the building blocks of proteins. It has many health benefits, it supports bones, joints, ligaments, and skin health. Both marrowbone and gelatine offer a wide range of health benefits when taken on a regular basis.

When my husband and I started sampling the desserts and other related food containing gelatine, remarkable things started happening, our nails grew longer without splitting, our skin seemed fresher, our hair seem to grow quickly, and other benefits happened with relation to our health. The most remarkable change I noticed, was the disappearance of the ache in my lower body and in my hip area when getting in and out of the car, and when doing other leg movements during my exercises.

Following is the extract taken from my recipe book: Devil Free Recipes.

Gelatine 'When adding gelatine to any recipe, buy pure, unflavoured 225 bloom gelatine. This is a high-grade product. If available, buy grass fed organic, beef gelatine. This gelatine cannot be obtained from any plant-based source. It is obtained from grass fed beef. Gelatine provides eight of the nine essential amino acids not synthesized by the human body but are essential to maintain good health. Gelatine promotes gut and digestive health, helps to maintain, and stabilise appetite which assists with healthy eating habits and reduces food cravings. It also helps with establishing weight control, assists with muscle recovery after exercise or injury; helps to develop strong bones, reduce pain and inflammation in joints; assists with hair and nail revitalisation and assists in developing a healthy immune system.'

I can only suggest you try gelatine for yourself. In doing so, do not buy any gelatine that has synthetic or food additive numbers on the ingredients panel at the side of the packaging. Do not buy any gelatine that has phosphate or phosphite added.

Now, it is time to get back to your last round of exercises for this book. Keeping in mind, that the next exercise involves lying on a soft carpet or exercise mat and the exercise will involve you getting down onto the floor to do this.

You may wish to wait until you are confident in your movements before tackling this one. Having said that, as your body becomes healthier, do not dismiss this exercise.

Regardless of how many exercises you have done in the past and how confident you feel, you may wish to do this exercise with another person in the room, it is always better to be safe than sorry!

LEG RAISING EXERCISE – USING YOUR QUADS TO BETTER HEALTH

Once lying on the carpet or exercise mat, and feeling comfortable, stretch both legs out straight without bending your knees.

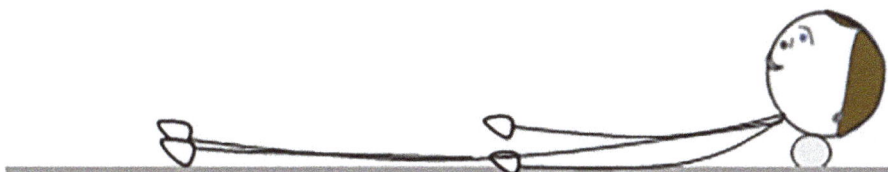

This exercise is great for firming up your calf muscles and quadriceps. Remember, your quads are the muscles that run along the side of the leg and connect to the knee. They absorb shock before it reaches your joints! This exercise will strengthen your knees and help to reduce pain and friction.

Once ready,

1. Lying on your back flat on the floor, keeping your knees straight, remember your breathing as you do the exercise.

2. Loosen your foot, now, with a little tension in your leg, keeping your knee straight, pull your toes towards you.

3. When you are ready, lift your foot up about six inches or (15cm), hold to the count of five. Lower your leg, rest, then repeat the exercise.

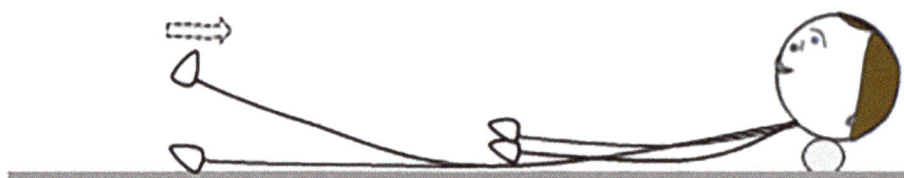

By doing this exercise every second day, you will be astonished at the improvement and strength in your knees. As your knees become stronger, and your confidence grows, you can add weights or heavier safe footwear to the exercise; this will add to the wellbeing of your knees, but only add extra weight when your knees are moving freely.

Always consult your health expert about the exercises you are undertaking.

GLUTE BRIDGING AND STRENGTHENING YOUR LOWER BODY

The glute bridge helps in exercising the whole of your lower half of your body. Remembering, your gluteal (glutes) muscles support the hip and leg muscles, (both your hips and legs have the ability to rotate inwards or outwards), this movement can only be done through the help of your glute muscles.

This exercise has all-round benefits. It supports your core becoming stronger, it helps in developing glute strength, strengthening hamstrings, and relieves pressure from your knee joints which helps you to keep your balance when walking and doing the things you want to do. This exercise helps to bring the enjoyment back into your life.

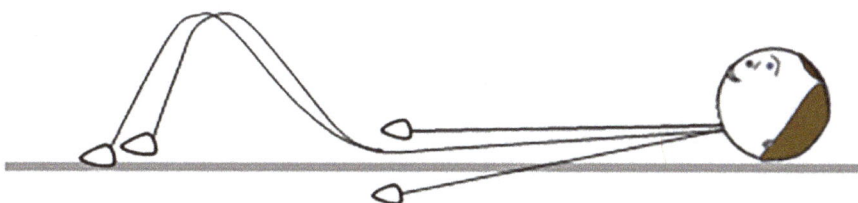

Staying in your lying position on the floor, remove the head support you have given yourself, lye flat but pull your knees up, keeping your feet firmly on the floor with your arms, and hands down by your sides; those too, resting on the floor.

1. Bring your feet in line with your hips.
2. Lift your bottom up as far as possible. As this is your first time, hold your position for as long as possible.
3. Lower your bottom and let it touch the floor. Take a short break and then do the exercise up to five times.

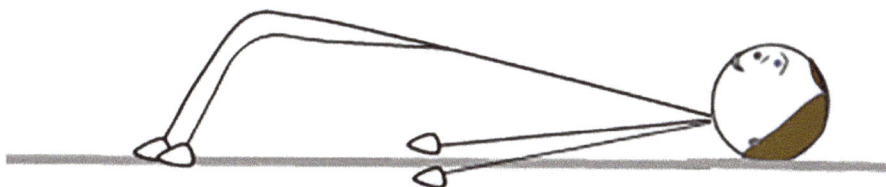

As your body loosens up and you are feeling confident about your exercises, you can extend the time and number of movements you want to achieve each time.

The release of tension within your muscles will start to lessen, through exercise you become more energetic, and your brain also feels the benefits because you will find your comprehension level increases and life in general becomes easier.

To help you achieve your fitness and health goals, please see, Grandma's Personal Trainer, Fitness Journal, now available.

SUMMARY OF MODULE FIVE

You have learnt:

✓ How gelatine and bone marrow can support you in gaining better health, freer movement, and wellbeing.

✓ You have gained the information that supports you in using your quadriceps that supports you in your knees and how using these muscles improves your overall good health and wellbeing.

✓ How using your gluteal (glutes) muscles help to support the hip and leg muscles, (both your hips and legs can rotate inwards or outwards). You now know that this movement is done through the support and help of your glute muscles.

CONGRATULATIONS – YOU HAVE FINISHED YOUR FIVE MODULES

'So, now, please keep your healthy regime alive by giving yourself the 'time out' to love and look after you.'

END OF MODULE FIVE

NOW AVAILABLE FOR YOU

'Grandma's Personal Trainer Goal Setting and Journal book.

Grandma's Personal Trainer Diary.

All are available at

www.how2books.com.au

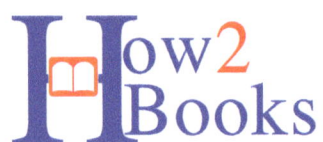

www.ingramcontent.com/pod-product-compliance
Lightning Source LLC
Chambersburg PA
CBHW060957030426
42334CB00032B/3274